Ultimate guide to Rapid Weight Loss Hypnosis

A Quick Guide To powerful weight loss method of using Guided Meditation and Affirmations for People Who Want Rapid Lose Weight, Increase Motivation and heal their body

Rihanna Smith

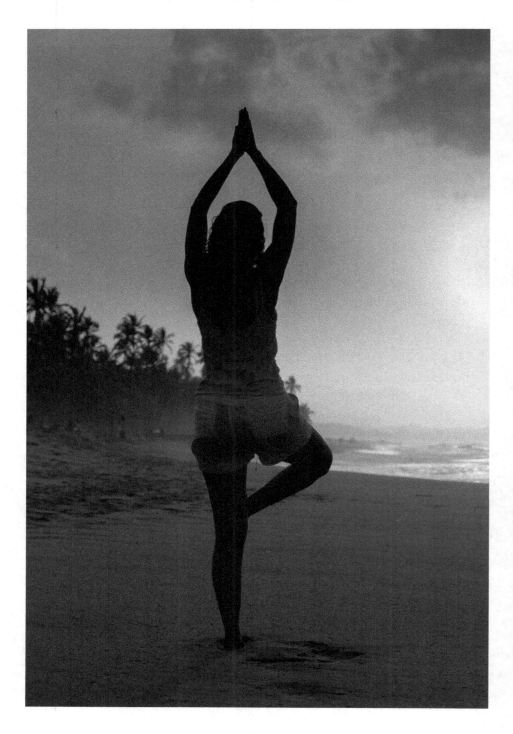

Table of Contents

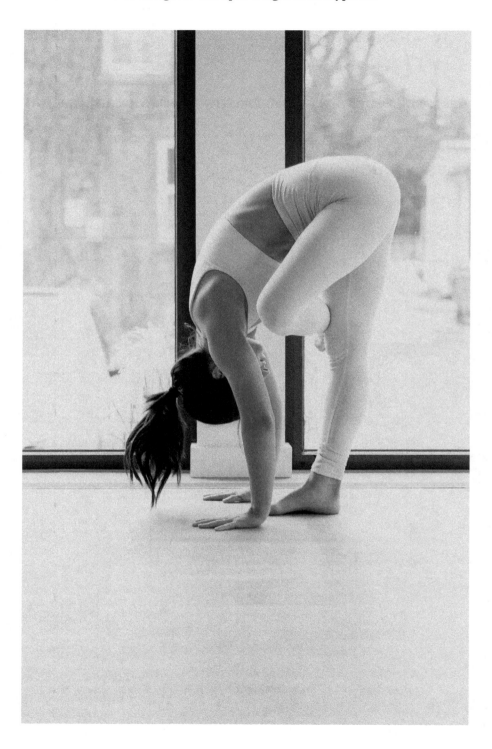

Introduction

The first thing you need to do is find that task you do not like. In some case there might be multiple of them depending on your personality and how you feel about your job. Now, try to look at why you do not like that task and do simple research on how to make the job a lot simpler. You can then start conditioning yourself to use the simple method every time you do the job.

After you are able to condition you state of mind to do the task, each time you encounter it will become the trigger for your trance and thus giving you the ability to perform it better. You will not be able to tell the difference since you will not mind it at all. Your coworkers and superiors though will definitely notice the change in your work style and in your productivity.

It is easy to improve in career. But to improve your relationship with you family can be a little trickier. Yet, self-hypnosis can still reprogram you to interact with your family members better by modifying how you react to the way they act. You will have the ability to adjust your way of thinking depending on the situation. This then allows you to respond in the most positive way possible no matter how dreadful the scenario may be.

If you are in a fight with your husband/wife for example, the normal reaction is to flare up and face fire with fire. The problem with this approach is it usually engulfs the entire relationship which might eventually lead up to separation. Being in a hypnotic state in this instance then can help you think clearly and change the impulse of saying words without thinking the through. Anger will still be there of course, that is the healthy way. But anger now under self-hypnosis can be channeled and stop being a raging inferno, you can turn it into a steady bonfire that can help you and your partner find common ground for whatever issue you are facing. The same applies in dealing with sibling or children. If you are able to condition your mind to think more rationally or to get into the perspective of others, then you can have better family/friends' relationships.

Losing weight can be the most common reason why people will use self-hypnosis in terms of health and physical activities. But this is just one part of it. Self-hypnosis can give you a lot more to improve this aspect of your life. It works the same way while working out.

Most people tend to give up their exercise program due to the exhaustion they think they can no longer take. But through self-hypnosis, you will be able to tell yourself that the exhaustion is lessened and thus allowing you to finish the entire routine. Keep in mind though that your mind must never be conditioned to forget exhaustion, it must only not mind it until the end of the exercise. Forgetting it completely might lead you to not stopping to work out until your energy is depleted. It becomes counterproductive in this case.

Having a healthy diet can also be influenced by self-hypnosis. Conditioning your mind to avoid unhealthy food can be done. Thus, hypnosis will be triggered each you are tempted to eat a meal you are conditioned to consider as unhealthy. Your eating habit then can change to benefit you to improve your overall health.

Mental, Emotional and Spiritual Needs

Since self-hypnosis deals directly in how you think, it is then no secret that it can greatly improve your mental, emotional and spiritual needs. A clear mind can give your brain the ability to have more rational thoughts. Rationality then leads to better decision making and easy absorption and retention of information you might need to improve your mental capacity. You must set your expectations though; this does not work like magic that can turn you into a genius. The process takes time depending on how far you are wanting to go, how much you want to achieve. Thus, the effects will only be limited by how much you are able to condition your mind.

In terms of emotional needs, self-hypnosis cannot make you feel differently in certain situations. But it can condition you to take in each scenario a little lighter and make you deal with them better. Others think that getting rid of emotion can be the best course of action if you are truly able to rewire your brain. But they seem to forget that even though rational thinking is often influenced negatively by emotion, it is still necessary for you to decide on things basing on the common ethics and aesthetics of the real world. Self-hypnosis then can channel your emotion to work in a more positive way in terms of decision making and dealing with emotional hurdles and problems.

Spiritual need on the other hand is far easier to influence when it comes to doing self-hypnosis. As a matter of fact, most people with spiritual beliefs are able to do self-hypnosis each time they practice what they believe in. A deep prayer for instance is a way to self-hypnotize yourself to enter the trance to feel closer to a Divine existence. Chanting and meditation done by other religions also leads and have the same goal. Even the songs during a mass or praise and worship triggers self-hypnosis depending if the person allows them to do so.

How hypnosis can help resolve childhood issues

Another issue that hypnosis can help is issues from our past. If you have had traumatic situations from your childhood days, then you may have issues in all areas of your adult life. Unresolved issues from your past can lead to anxiety and depression in your later years. Childhood trauma is dangerous because it can alter many things in the brain both psychologically and chemically.

The most vital thing to remember about trauma from your childhood is that given a harmless and caring environment in which the child's vital needs for physical safety, importance, emotional security and attention are met, the damage that trauma and abuse cause can be eased and relieved. Safe and dependable relationships are also a dynamic component in healing the effects of childhood trauma in adulthood and make an atmosphere in which the brain can safely start the process of recovery.

There is a deeper realism active at all times around us and inside us. This reality commands that we must come to this world to find happiness, and every so often that our inner child stands in our way. This is by no means intentional; however, it desires to reconcile wounds from the past or address damaging philosophies which were troubling to us as children.

So to disengage the issues that upset us from earlier in our lives we have to find a way to bond with our internal child, we then need to assist in rebuilding this part of us which will in turn help us to be rid of all that has been hindering us from moving on.

Breathe in and loosen your clothing if you have to. Inhale deeply into your abdomen and exhale, repeat until you feel yourself getting relaxed; you may close your eyes and focus on getting less tense. Feel your forehead and head relax, let your face become relaxed and relax your shoulders. Allow your body to be limp and loose while you breathe slowly. Keep breathing slowly as you let all of your tension float away.

Now slowly count from 10-0 in your mind and try to think of a place from your childhood. The image doesn't have to be crystal clear right now but try to focus on exactly how you remember it and keep that image in mind. Imagine yourself as a child and imagine observing younger you; think about your clothes, expression, hair etc. In your mind go and meet yourself, introduce yourself to you.

CHAPTER 1:

Increase Your Motivation

The first thing you are going to want to do to motivate you is to change your attitude into a positive one. When we look at the world through a grey lens, we can easily see everything as terrible. When you hate one thing, that hate starts to grow and can spread into other parts of your life. We can't look at life through rose-colored glasses either, because we don't want to make ourselves ignorant to reality. We have to look at the world, at our life, head-on, as it is objectively. When we can do this, it will be much easier to take on the new things that present themselves to you every day.

Give yourself time to prepare to be motivated too, not just time to start the weight loss. First, you have to get in the right mindset. Then, you can prepare for your meal plan and exercise regimen before starting. If you try to force yourself into it, you might sometimes make it even harder to get started.

As humans, we like to be independent. Not everyone is interested in being told what to do, and we sometimes seek to be defiant in ways, even against ourselves. Sometimes in our heads, the things we're being told to do won't be our ideas and can instead be the pressures of society, our peers, and our parents. Their voices can still get so deep in our heads that we will mistake them for our own and can easily get frustrated with what we're telling ourselves.

It can seem like an internal battle when you are trying to get motivated. There's the part of you that knows what you have to do, and then there's the voice that's telling you not to do it. To sit around and wait for tomorrow. Motivation is all about silencing that voice and building one of encouragement.

You are the person that you are right now because of the life that you've lived. It can be so easy to think, "Oh, I should have done this," or "if only I had gone with the other option." However, if we hadn't made that one choice, then our lives would be incredibly different than what they are now. Each thing we've experienced, the decisions we've made, and the thoughts that we've had, these are all like ingredients that go into what makes us who we are. When you can learn to love yourself and the person that you've become, then it will be easier to build that motivation because you'll let that guilt and regret losing.

Look at what motivates you right now, at this very second. What's the first thing that comes to mind? Maybe it is wanting to make a loved one proud or providing for your child. Perhaps your motivation is getting your bills paid or merely making your next meal. Whatever it is, this can tell you a lot about what drives you in this life. When you can become aware of all the motivating factors in your life, it will be a lot easier to use these images and ideas when you are struggling in certain situations. If nothing comes to mind at all, then it is time to do some soul searching. At the very least, wanting to make ourselves happy should be a motivator. Feeling good and looking better is all I need to motivate me on some days; however, others require a little more work.

Honestly, sometimes food was a motivator for me. I would tell myself that if I could avoid fast food all week and eat healthy Monday-Friday, that Saturday, I could go crazy. I told myself it didn't' matter if I wanted to drive myself through Taco Bell, Wendy's, and KFC all in one week. Whatever I decided for Saturday would be fine, as long as I stayed resilient against my cravings for Monday-Friday. If I was struggling on Wednesday and just wanted to skip the salad I brought to work and walk to the fast-food joint across the street; I would remind myself that I could get it on Saturday. When I would diet in the past, I would think that I had to cut all lousy food out for the time being. It would drive me crazy!

What would end up happening was that I felt so good about myself for eating healthy all week that I wouldn't want to ruin my streak so I would keep up the diet. I would get to Saturday and think to myself that I had done so well all week, why ruin it now? I might still occasionally go out to dinner with my family on the weekends and get something that isn't great for me, but then this was a reward. I realized that motivation would breed more motivation.

The easier it was for me to get started with the things I want and stay focused on my goals, the more this strengthened my willpower. There are always going to be hard days, but I just remind myself that this is part of the process.

Research on Motivation

We need the motivation to do anything. A lot of times, we don't realize the motivation behind specific actions. How many times have you reflected on something you've done and thought, "Why on Earth did I just do that?" Though we feel like we're in charge often, there are a lot of times when it feels like we have almost no control at all. This is because sometimes, our subconscious will think it knows what's best for us better than we would of ourselves. The better we can understand our motivation on an individual level, the easier it will be to create those feelings of encouragement within ourselves. Those that struggle with weight loss aren't the only ones who are concerned with motivation either. Since it is so relevant in all aspects of life, we have scientific research that allows us insight into what might drive our most basic desires.

We have two different kinds of goals when it comes to motivation, mastery and performance5. On the one hand, you might desire to achieve something because you want to master that task.

Your Reason for Motivation

Finding a solid reason to lose weight is something that's going to be very important in your journey. On the one hand, you won't want to do it just for other people. This is something that you have to do for yourself. If you're going to make your spouse, children, peers, parents, or anyone else proud, that's great! But you have to remember that what will matter most in this journey is making yourself proud.

Competition can be helpful, but at first, you just need to focus on yourself, especially if this has been a long journey for you. If you're too competitive, then you might make yourself feel bad. Competition should be fun and encouraging, like doing a small race with a friend. If you base your life around it and only find worth in beating other people, then that's going to be harmful to your perspective on yourself, making it even more challenging to lose the weight and keep it off.

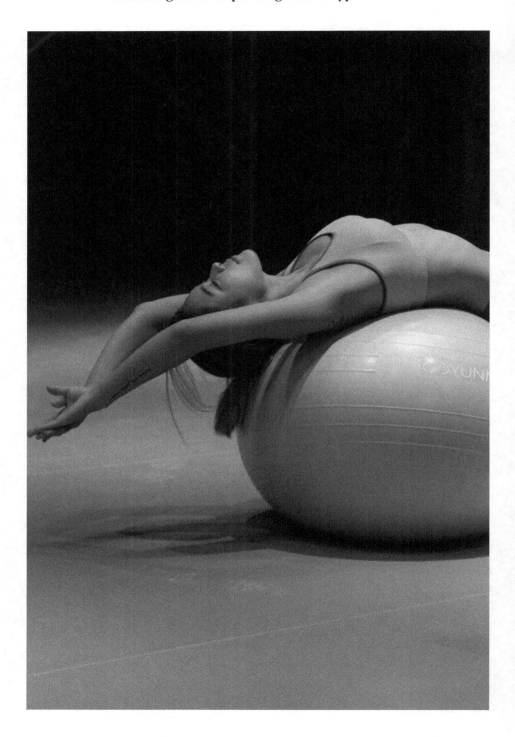

CHAPTER 2:

Losing Weight With Hypnosis:
A Real Replacement for Diet

Weight loss due to hypnosis-sounds like a dream for Martina S. She already had a long diet odyssey behind her. She failed with FdH, combined meals, dieted, and slimmed drinks. After she finally approached her ideal weight with Weight Watchers, the pound returned to her waist after the program.

Weight loss due to hypnosis

Then she read a daily newspaper ad: "Hypnotizing to the desired weight-simple, permanent, without willpower and meals." Then she got new hope. With a price of 100 euros in a one-off session and a promised success rate of 80%, we dare to make a relatively realistic female attempt in other respects. In a few days, 12 practice in beach chair advertising practitioners practice. In addition to being overweight, it is in Schleswig-Holstein. "I was relatively excited before, but this session had nothing to do with the show Hypnose hype on TV.

Like snoozing in the sun

"Since then, the actual transformer treatment has begun," the nurse says. During hypnosis, she felt as relaxed as when she fell asleep in the sun. "In the distance, I heard the therapist say that I will eat when I am hungry. Martina says I will not eat after 6 pm." Today, three months later, a scale Is about 15 kilometers less, and Martina's desire for sweets is not overwhelming. "It's almost scary, but there is no desire for chocolate or fatty food. Even colleagues have already realized that they can't even reach their nostrils automatically." Work?

Example of a case of Weight Loss by Hypnosis

An overweight woman asked me for help in controlling her diet. His problem was a compulsion to eat popcorn. He bought them in packages of 45 kilos, ate popcorn with butter at all hours, and quench his thirst; he drank copious amounts of soda. Butter, salt, and soda were more harmful to her than popcorn, although they represented the vehicle for ingesting the other products. So it was appropriate to make popcorn, not to your liking.

Before I hypnotized her, I tried to discover what foods she didn't like, but she seemed to like everything.

"Is there nothing that you find repulsive?" I asked the edge of despair.

"Well, yes," he replied. «The wet feathers of chickens make me sick. I can't stand his smell. My father forced me to kill and peel chickens against my will. I had finally found something wet chicken feathers. When we practiced exercise J, and we reached the moment when she should put something in her mouth, I said: "There is a large bowl full of popcorn in front of you, but they have been in contact with wet chicken feathers. Popcorn smells like feathers. Now take a handful of popcorn and place it in your mouth. He immediately began to gag and feel nauseous. I thought I was about to throw up.

When he left the office and arrived at his house, he prepared some popcorn. It was then that he vomited. Every day he tried to eat popcorn, but the mere fact of preparing them made him nauseous. When he returned to the office for the third session, he was not even trying to develop the popcorn he had abandoned the habit and was losing weight. When he stopped eating popcorn, he also left soda, butter, and salt.

When we were approaching session number 6, I had already lost almost 9 kilos and felt very good. I told him to add more fruit and vegetables to the diet. I had stopped being a popcorn addict.

The lesson we must learn from this example is that it is necessary to discover some taste or smell that is repulsive to the patient. Such flavors or odors will be used later to eliminate a harmful habit. Most often, the problem is sweets, such as chocolate or cakes. If the subject drinks 51 pounds (2 kilos) of chocolate a day and hates the taste of the liver, he should instruct to visualize himself removing a piece of chocolate from the fridge that has been very close to a part of 2 kilos of the fresh liver The taste and smell of the liver have permeated chocolate you can get an idea.

Exercises before Hypnosis

. - Below, I will present two exercises before hypnosis. You must use them during the consultation period to become familiar with hypnosis and to feel comfortable. Words written in italics indicate the text that should be said aloud.

Exercise 1:

I want you to close your eyes for a short workout. I want you to imagine a blackboard, to believe it. It can be black or green, or the color you want. Believe it, The board has a tray, and there are chalk and an eraser on it. Do you see her?

(Wait for the answer. When the subject answers affirmatively, you can continue.)

Very well. Now take chalk and draw a circle on the board. Have you brought it yet?

Good. Now write the letter A inside the circle. Have you done it yet?

Now you delete the letter A inside the circle but do not remove the ring. Let me know when you're done.

(Wait for the answer).

Very good. Now erase the circle and open your eyes.

At this point, you can briefly talk with the patient about the experience of the board. Assure him that whatever knowledge he has had, it has been positive. Each person responds differently. Some see the board. Others intuit it. Some know that it is there. All the answers are correct. In hypnosis, there are no erroneous experiences; Each person lives the situations in a personal way, and all the skills are valid. Clarify to the patient that these types of responses are frequent in hypnosis.

Exercise 2:

Close your eyes once again to perform another training exercise. This time I want him to focus his attention on the tip of his nose. Has it done?

Wait for the affirmative answer, and continue.

All right. Keep your attention on the tip of the nose and listen to the sound of my voice, in some of the hypnosis techniques that we will do together. If at any time during hypnosis, you warn that your mind wanders, all you have to do is focus again on the tip of your nose just as you are doing right now. Then your account will stop wavering and concentrate on my voice again. Now you can open your eyes.

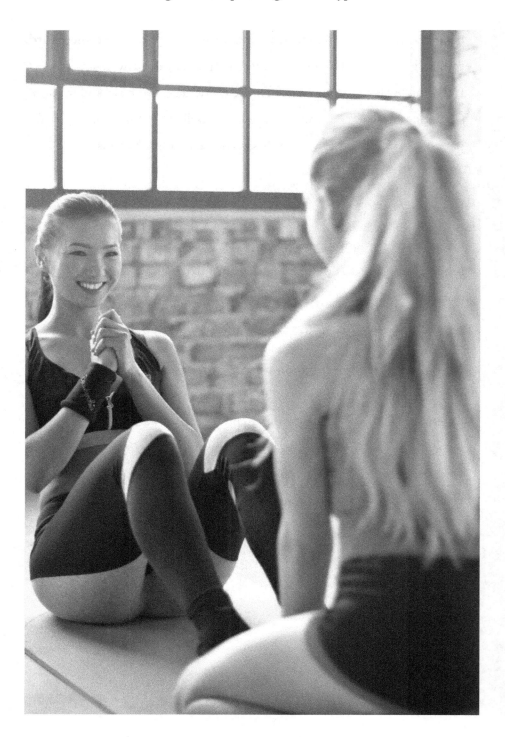

CHAPTER 3:

Self Hypnosis

A Few Simple Rules

There are a few guidelines to hypnosis, and they guarantee that your training is the most proficient and yields the best advantages. At the point when you are prepared to start utilizing the sound, locate an agreeable and safe spot in your home or office where you can sit in a seat, lean back, or even rests. Ensure you are loose and in a spot where you don't need to focus on whatever else. Try not to tune in to your daze work while you are driving a vehicle or working any kind of hardware. It is useful to settle on a customary time every day or night to rehearse your self-hypnosis. Sleep time is a decent chance to make the most of your stupor work, and rehearsing as of now can be a great method to enter a tranquil sleep.

Interruptions and interferences are unavoidable. As opposed to permitting them to bother you and remove you from your stupor work, use them. Utilize the sounds in the earth around you to improve your daze understanding. For instance, while doing your hypnosis, you may see a sound and begin imagining that this sound is diverting you. You, at that point, become more centered on this interruption than on your hypnosis. You might be enticed to battle against it—which removes vitality from the hypnosis. Rather, when you notice a sound that from the outset appears diverting or irritating, assume responsibility for it by giving it your authorization to be there as a foundation sound. Give it a task, for example, contemplating internally that "the sound of the yapping hound is helping me go deeper and deeper inside" or "the fan engine seems like a cascade that is an alleviating foundation sound." At our private practice in Tucson, there is a day school that unavoidably lets the youngsters out to play during one of our hypnosis meetings. That is the point at which we recommend, "The sound of youngsters can be a foundation sound that releases you deeper and deeper inside yourself now." This is a piece of our "utilization everything" theory.

Law of Reversed Effect

There is a law in hypnosis, called the Law of Reversed Effect, that says that occasionally the more you attempt to accomplish something, the more it doesn't occur. A model is a point at which you need to state a name that you realize, you know—it might be a book title, an individual, a film—however, you can't state it at that point, and the more you attempt, the less it is there. The name comes when you propose to your subconscious mind that "I'll recollect later" or "It'll come to me later." By relinquishing the inquiry, "What's the name? What's the name?" you have discharged your subconscious mind to now recover and convey the appropriate response, and it generally does. Along these lines, the Law of Reversed Effect is that when you are making a decent attempt for something, it just gives you the inverse (the opposite).

Basic Techniques

Getting ingested in your considerations and thoughts is that delicate excursion into the focal point of you called "going into a stupor." The straightforward methods of self-hypnosis incorporate going into a daze, deepening the daze, utilizing that daze state to give messages and recommendations to the mind-body, and coming out of the daze.

Subconscious Mind (Or Unconscious Mind)

This is the bit of our mind that performs capacities and procedures beneath our reasoning mindfulness. It is the mind of the body. It inhales us, digests, beats our hearts, and as a rule, deals with our automatic physical procedures for us. It can likewise instruct us to pick a bit of new mango rather than chocolate cake, to quit eating when we are full, or to appreciate a stroll in the recreation center.

Going into Trance

At the point when you are utilizing the stupor take a shot at the sound, I will be your guide as you go into a daze. I will utilize a daze enlistment strategy that you will discover quieting and centering. You have most likely observed the swinging watch technique in motion pictures, which is thirty-five years of training I have never observed anybody use, yet there is a wide range of approaches to concentrate on going into a stupor. You may gaze at a spot on the divider, utilize a breathing procedure, or utilize dynamic body unwinding. You will hear an assortment of acceptance strategies on the stupor work sound. They are just the prompts or the signs that you are providing for yourself to state, "I am going into a daze" or "I will do my hypnosis currently." Going into stupor can likewise be thought of as "letting yourself dream … intentionally."

You are letting yourself become consumed in your contemplations and thoughts, exceptionally ingested, and permitting yourself to imagine or envision what you want as accomplished and genuine. There is no "going under." Instead, there is a beautiful encounter of going inside.

Deepening the Trance

Deepening your stupor causes you to become increasingly invested in your contemplations, thoughts, and experience. This is finished with dynamic unwinding: going "deeper and deeper inside …" with pictures or scenes, or by checking a number arrangement, for instance. We like to propose that as you hear the checking from ten to zero, you make a vertical symbolism that is related to going deeper, for example, a way driving da mountain or into a rich green valley.

As you hear me tallying, you can picture or envision going all the more deeply into a scene or spot that is considerably progressively pleasant and agreeable to you. This is the thing that we mean by "deepening the stupor."

Cognizant Mind

This is the "thinking mind" or the piece of the mind that gives us our mindfulness or feeling of knowing and oversees our deliberate capacities. For instance, our cognizant mind takes that second bit of pie at the meal, swipes the check card at the market, and moves the fork to our mouth.

Conversing with The Mind of Your Body with Messages and Suggestions

During the day's work, you will hear my voice addressing two pieces of your mind. One piece of your mind is your cognizant reasoning mind. That is the piece of you that is phenomenal at reading a clock, making change, figuring out how to peruse, and compose; it is your "thinking mind." Throughout the day's work, your reasoning mind will keep doing its typical action of having musings. So, you don't need to stress over clearing your mind, or exhausting your mind, or putting your mind settled. Essentially notice that your mind will keep "thinking and your main responsibility is to unplug or detach simply enough with the goal that you don't need to respond to those contemplations. You give them consent to stream by. If your schedule keeps springing up, for instance, simply permit it to stream by, as opposed to harp on it.

The other piece of your mind I will be addressing is the thing that we call your subconscious mind—"sub" since it is beneath your considering level mindfulness. It is the "mind of your body." Your subconscious mind has the astuteness to deal with your body's trillions of cells, your body science, and all the body's elements of breathing, absorption, the sensory system, the endocrine framework, and the resistant framework. The mind-body has a huge measure of knowledge, and, in doing your hypnosis, you are gathering and obtaining extra insight that the mind of your body will follow up on, predictable with your motivation, your convictions, and your desires, to assist you with your weight loss.

You generally have the chance to alter and tailor the words being verbally expressed or the pictures portrayed to best fit you. This fitting procedure is significant. It needs to fit you, since it is your self-hypnosis, and all hypnosis is self-hypnosis. As we've stated, hypnosis isn't something done to you. It is something that you are being guided to understanding, and as you experience it, you are learning it. Repetition and practice make strong capacity and information inside you. You may even call it subconscious information because your subconscious mind can do it for you without your night consider it. So the musings and thoughts that may have been alarming you about your weight, or your failure to get more fit, are presently being changed to something that bolsters your ideal body. What's more, your mind-body is retaining the experience with the goal that it can allude to that understanding rather than the undesirable consequences of the past.

For instance, if you accept that you are a "yo-yo" dieter since you have consistently recaptured the weight you have lost, you may utilize your trancework to propose, "Each day I am getting in shape, and my body recalls how to make this a perpetual capacity. I am accomplishing my

31

ideal weight." Subconscious information, or the mind-body intelligence that is found out from your trance work, is especially similar to when you figured out how to ride a bike or drive a vehicle. At the point when you were first learning, there appeared to be numerous things to focus on simultaneously, however rapidly your mind-body took on this information with the goal that now you can drive securely. You don't need to instruct your feet.

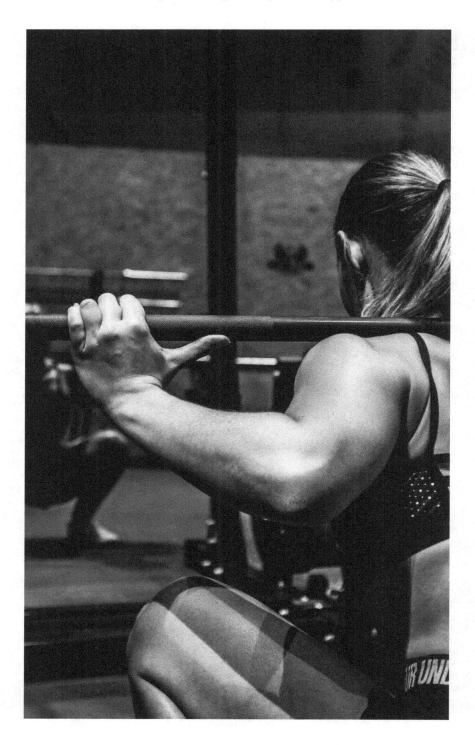

CHAPTER 4:

Essential Ingredients to
Make Self-Hypnosis Work

Disclaimer: Before you start listening make sure that you are in a quiet room, away from any distractions, and please use headphones.

This technique is based on the power of self-hypnosis to strengthen your motivation in planning a healthy weight loss.

(put music with binaural sounds)

Close your eyes.

—

Make contact with the breath.

Allow my voice to guide you through this process.

—

Inhale through your nostrils, mentally counting to three.

One.

Two.

Three.

Hold your breath.

Exhale from the nostrils, mentally counting to four.

One.

Two.

Three.

Four.

—

By following the sound of my voice, you will relax more and more.

—

Let your attention sink, as if you had thrown a pebble into a lake and watched it go down into the depths of the waters.

—

Deeper and deeper, in the quiet blue waters of relaxation.

—

Feel the relaxation of the shoulders, the heaviness of the arms.

—

Your breathing becomes deeper and deeper, the muscles of the face are relaxed.

—

You are relaxing more and more, you are sliding to a level of total abandonment.

—

You are already changing, with your commitment to lose weight, to stay fit and healthy, for a lifetime.

—

Yes, you are much better when you feel good in your body.

—

Feel the euphoria grow for your lean and healthy body. It is the same euphoria you feel in front of an unexpected gift.

The more you discard the gift, the more you feel joy.

Let this joy grow.

—

As I count from five to one, you relax more and more and you feel determined to achieve your goals.

—

It is time to command a change within you, which will allow you to make wiser and healthier choices regarding the care of your body and your health.

—

Five.

You know why you want this change: being fit will make you feel good.

—

Four.

Being fit will improve your life,

your job,

your relationships,

your self-confidence.

Being fit will make you feel good.

—

Three.

Open the gift of the future, in the present, now. See yourself as you want to be: see the self of the future now, in the present. Fit and healthy, slim and happy.

—

Two.

Observe the expression on the face of that future yourself: she is relaxed, determined, focused. That's right, just like that.

—

One.

Relax completely now.

—

There is no need to make any effort: your mind will listen and make sense of these words.

—

Now give your body a new lifestyle.

A lifestyle that chooses healthy foods and regular exercise.

Who chooses sunlight and fresh air?

Who chooses to be fit, beautiful and healthy?

—

Here, you become thin, beautiful and healthy as you were born to be.

—

Remember the great goal you want to achieve: lose weight, make your body healthier and stay fit.

—

Focus on the future you want for yourself. The future in which you are thin, beautiful and healthy.

The future in which you release well-being, charm and joie de vivre

—

Take a step towards that future yourself, get closer to who you want to become.

—

Enter that future yourself now.

Feel your determination, your commitment to take care of your body, to nourish it always at its best.

—

Feel how your future self is already helping you now, how an adult helps a child avoid dangers, and teaches him what's best for him.

—

Bring your future self into the present yourself.

Now bring what you want to be into what you are.

—

Spread your arms in front of you. Keep them straight in front of you.

Let your mind bring your arms together automatically.

—

The closer the arms come the more your lean, beautiful, healthy body enters your body now.

—

The closer the arms come, the more your lean, beautiful, healthy body becomes your body now.

—

The closer the arms come, the more what you want to become becomes what you already are.

—

Let your arms come automatically together.

—

When your hands have joined together, feel the well-being of your lean, beautiful, healthy body within you.

—

When the hands come together, you have completed the process: you have brought your new body into your body.

—

When the hands come together, stay in this position and see your new body.

—

Listen to your new body.

—

Feel your new body.

—

Then bring your arms back to your sides.

—

You brought your new body inside you.

—

Feel the pride and joy of having this new body.

—

With this new skinny body, you are now walking.

—

You walk with your new skinny body around the city and you feel perfectly at ease.

You feel confident.

Do you feel OK.

—

Meet your friends and hear their compliments on your fitness.

—

Everyone compliments you because you have become what you wanted to become.

—

Your future body is already your body. Just now.

—

Bring your new body into your daily life.

—

Day after day, you will get closer and closer to your new body.

—

Day after day, you will become your new body more and more.

—

Day after day, you will be increasingly motivated to lose weight.

—

You are about to return to the waking state.

Get ready to bring this new body into your waking state.

—

Your subconscious mind will process every word I said and you listened.

—

Every time you hear these words, the suggestion will become more and more powerful for you.

—

Whenever you hear these words, the suggestion will become an increasingly important part of you.

Every time you listen to these words, you will become more and more the person you have chosen to be.

I will count from one to five and at the end of the count you will feel completely awake and better than before.

—

One.

Feel a nice feeling of lightness and peace. You feel increasingly motivated to lose weight.

Two.

You will maintain the resolve and determination within you every day. You feel even more motivated to lose weight.

Three.

In a very short time, you will wake up and you will be even more motivated to lose weight.

Four.

You feel perfectly awake, ready to return to the present and motivated to lose weight.

Five.

Open your eyes.

Welcome back.

(turn off the music with binaural sounds)

CHAPTER 5:

Overcoming Negative Habits

The longer the habit we have with us, the more often we do it, the more secure it will be, and the harder it will be to wipe it off. Please quit overeating. It is not uncommon to start eating without knowing it when already taken a full meal or when absorbed in conversation or work.

Such habits have physical-neurologic-foundation. The neural pathways in our body can be compared to unpaved roads. This road is smooth before vehicles drive on dirt roads. When a car first rides on the road, its tires leave marks, but the ruts are flat. Rain and wind can easily pass by and smooth the road again. However, after 100 rides with deeper and deeper tires, rain and wind make little impression on the deep ruts. They stay there.

The same applies to people. To expand the metaphor a little, we were born with a smooth street in our heads. When a young child first buttons a jacket or ties a shoe, the effort is tedious, clumsy, and frustrating. More trials are needed until the child gets the hang of it, and a successful move becomes a behavioral pattern.

From a physiological point of view, these movement instructions travel along nerve paths to the muscles and back again. The message is sent to the central nervous system along an afferent pathway. The "I want to lift my legs" impulse continues in the efferent pathway from the central nervous system to my muscles: "Raise my legs." After a while, such messages are automatically enriched by countless repetitions and automatically sent at electrical speed.

Return to the car and the street. Suppose the car decides to avoid a worn groove and take a new path. What's going on the car will go straight back into the old ditch. Like people trying to get out of old habits, they tend to revert to old habits.

Still, we haven't developed any unwanted habits. We learn them, and we can rewind the learning. It can be unconditional. And here, self-hypnosis takes place, pushing the individual out of the established habit gap in a smooth manner of new behavior.

The advantage it offers compared to simple willpower trial and error results from an increase in the state of consciousness that characterizes the state of self-hypnosis. A further extension of the unpaved road analogy is that the hovercraft slides a few centimeters above the road, over a rut or habit. Regardless of the habit of working, the implementation process is the same.

Only the verbal implant and the image below are different. To encapsulate the induction process, count one, for one thing, two for two things and count three for three things:

1. Please raise your eyes as high as possible.

2. Still staring, slowly close your eyes and take a deep breath.

3. Exhale, relax your eyes, and float your body. Then, if time permits, spend a little more time and introduce yourself to the most comfortable, calm, and pleasant place in your imagination.

Now, when you float deep inside the resting chair, you will feel a little away from your body. It's another matter, so you can give her instructions on how to behave.

At this point, the specific purpose of self-hypnosis determines the expression and image content of the syllogism. It provides suggestions for discussing different habits that can be followed as shown or modified as needed. This strategy can help overcome the habit of overeating.

Overall, we are a country boasting abundant food. Most of us (with the blatant and lamentable exception) have enough money to make sure we are comfortably overeating. As a result, many of us get obese. So, the weight loss business is a big industry. Tablet makers, diet developers, and exercise studios will not confuse customers who want to lose weight.

It is said that every fat person who has a hard time escaping has lost weight. Unfortunately, too often, the lean man spends his life, nevertheless never succeeding in his escape. Despite the image of a funny fat man, everyone rarely enjoys being overweight-most people become unhappy, rarely so confident, and less than confident and ruining their lives. Obesity seems to creep on only some of us, and by the time we notice it, it is a painful habit to overeat or eat, like the excess weight itself.

Self-hypnosis can help this lean man release his bond of "too hard" and start a new life. An article in the International Journal of Clinical and Experimental Hypnosis (January 1975) reports on such cases. Sidney E. and Mitchell P. Pulver cite family doctors study hypnosis in medical and dental practice.

Dr. Roger Bernhardt, while mentioning one of his overweight patients, said that "I brought the patient to the hospital for about a year and a half ago. She went to many doctors to cut back. She said she was rarely leaving home because she was extremely obese; she was relaxing and avoiding people. She came in for £ 380. I started trans in my first session. She continued on a diet and focused on telling her she would like people when she lost weight. She came for the first three or four sessions each week, after which

I started teaching her self-hypnosis. Now, this woman lost a total of £ 150, but beyond that, she became another person. She was virtually introverted and rarely came out of her home. She dared to do a part-time job in cosmetics. She hosts a party to show off her cosmetics and hypnotizes herself before the party. She became the state's second-largest saleswoman and earned tens of thousands of dollars."

Simply put, here are the therapies you should use when using self-hypnosis for weight management. After provoking self-hypnosis, mentally recite the syllogism. "I need my body alive. To the extent I want to live, I protect my body just as I protect it."

In the case of a tie mate picture, one can imagine himself in two situations where he is likely to overeat: between meals and at the dining table. With his eyes closed, he imagines a movie screen on the wall. He is on the screen himself, in every situation he finds when he is reading, chatting with others, watching TV, or having trouble calorie counting.

The second scene that catches your eye is the dining table. Do you tend to grab this second loaf? Instead, put your hand on your forehead and remember, "Protect my body." Looking at a cake, a loaf, a potato, or a cake raises the idea, "This is for someone. I'm good enough". With the fork down, take a deep breath and be proud to help one-person flow through the body.

Then, imagine a very simple and effective exercise method that simply puts your hand on the edge of the table and pushes it. Better yet, stand up from the chair and leave the table at this point.

Here's another image I'd recommend to a self-hypnotist. If you introduce yourself to the screen of this fictional movie, you will find yourself slim. Give yourself the ideal line that you want to see to others. Cut the abdomen and waistline to the desired ratio. Take an imaginary black pencil, sketch the entire picture, and make the lines sharp and solid. Hold photo because you can keep this slender picture, you can lose weight.

Then get out of your hypnosis and repeat it regularly every few hours. Exercise is especially useful during the temptation to be used as a comfortable, calorie-free substitute for fatty snacks or as an additional serving with meals. It would be a good time to practice it just before dinner.

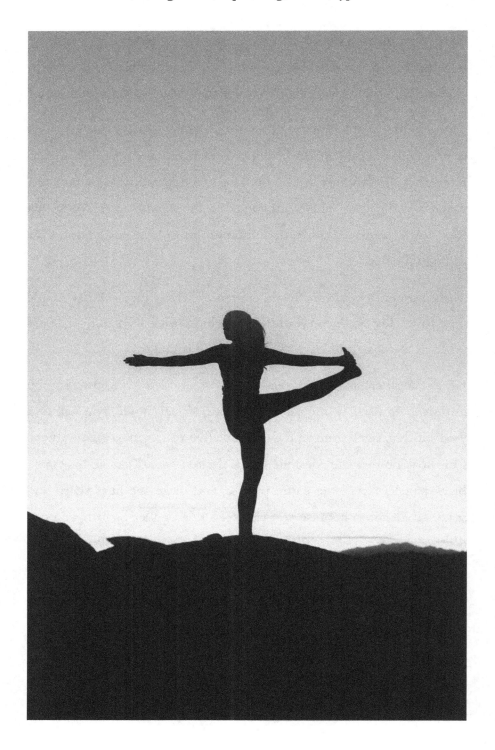

CHAPTER 6:

Daily Habits for Weight Loss

My careful eating procedure is figuring out how to be cautious. Rather than eating carelessly, putting nourishment unknowingly in your mouth, not tasting the sustenance you eat, you see your thoughts, and feelings.

- Learn to be cautious: why you want to eat, and what emotions or requirements can trigger eating.
- What you eat, and whether it's reliable.
- Look, smell, taste; feel the nourishment that you eat.
- How do you feel when you taste it, how would you digest it, and go about your day?
- How complete you are previously, during, and in the wake of eating.
- During and in the wake of eating, your sentiments.
- Where the nourishment originated from, who could have developed it, the amount it could have suffered before it killed, whether it naturally developed, the amount it was handled, the amount it was broiled or overcooked, and so on.

This is an ability that you don't merely increase medium-term, a type of reflection. It takes practice, and there will be times when you neglect to eat mindfully, begin, and stop. However, you can generally get excellent at this with exercise and consideration.

Mindful Eating Benefits

The upsides of eating are unimaginable, and realizing these points of interest is fundamental as you think about the activity.

· When you're anxious, you figure out how to eat and stop when you're plunking down.

· You figure out how to taste nourishment and acknowledge great sustenance tastes.

· You start to see that unfortunate nourishment isn't as delicious as you accepted, nor does it make you feel extremely pleasant.

· Because of the over three points, if you are overweight, you will regularly get more fit.

· You start arranging your nourishment and eating through the passionate issues you have. It requires somewhat more, yet it's essential.

· Social overeating can turn out to be less of an issue—you can eat while mingling, rehearsing, and not over-alimenting.

· You begin to appreciate the experience of eating more, and as an outcome, you will acknowledge life more when you are progressively present.

· It can transform into a custom of mindfulness that you anticipate.

· You learn for the day how nourishment impacts your disposition and vitality.

· You realize what fuel your training best with nourishment, and you work and play.

A Guide to Mindful Eating

Keeping up a contemporary, quick-paced way of life can leave a brief period to oblige your necessities. You are moving always starting with one thing then onto the next, not focusing on what your psyche or body truly needs. Rehearsing mindfulness can help you to comprehend those necessities.

When eating mindfulness is connected, it can help you recognize your examples and practices while simultaneously standing out to appetite and completion related to body signs.

You were originating from the act of pressure decrease dependent on mindfulness, rehearsing mindfulness. At the same time, eating can help you focus on the present minute instead of proceeding with ongoing and unacceptable propensities.

Careful eating is an approach to begin an internal looking course to help you become increasingly aware of your nourishment association and utilize that information to eat with joy.

The body conveys a great deal of information and information, so you can start settling on conscious choices instead of falling into programmed — and regularly feeling driven — practices when you apply attention to the eating knowledge. You are better prepared to change your conduct once you become aware of these propensities.

Individuals that need to be cautious about sustenance and nourishment are asked to:

· Explore their inward knowledge about food—different preferences

· Choose sustenance that pleases and support their bodies

· Accept explicit sustenance inclinations without judgment or self-analysis

General Principles of Mindful Eating

One methodology to careful eating depends on the core values given by Rebecca J. Frey, Ph.D., and Laura Jean Cataldo, RN: tune in to the internal craving and satiety signs of your body Identify own triggers for careless eating, for example, social weights, incredible sentiments, and explicit nourishments.

Here are a couple of tips for getting you started.

· Start with one meal. It requires some investment to begin with any new propensity. It very well may be challenging to make cautious eating rehearses regularly. However, you can practice with one dinner or even a segment of a supper. Attempt to focus on appetite sign and sustenance choices before you start eating or sinking into the feelings of satiety toward the part of the arrangement—these are unique approaches to begin a routine with regards to consideration.

· Remove view distractions place or turn off your phone in another space. Mood killers such as the TV and PC and set away whatever else —, for example, books, magazines, and papers—that can divert you from eating. Give the feast before your complete consideration.

· Tune in your perspective when you start this activity, become aware of your attitude. Perceive that there is no right or off base method for eating, yet only unmistakable degrees of eating background awareness. Focus your consideration on eating sensations. When you understand that your brain has meandered, take it delicately back to the eating knowledge.

· Take as much time as necessary. Eating includes backing off, enabling your stomach related hormones to tell your mind that you are finished before overeating. It's a fabulous method to hinder your fork between chomps. Additionally, you will be better prepared to value your supper experience, especially if you're with friends and family.

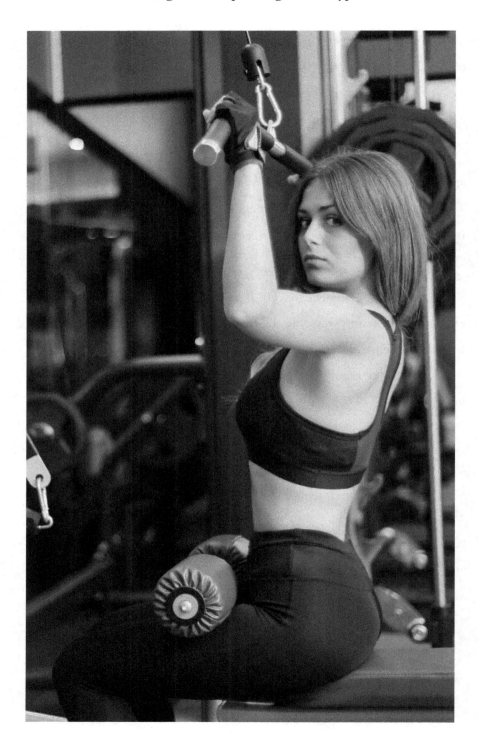

CHAPTER 7:

Mindful Eating Habits

When was the last time you went to the market with the intention of specifically buying fruits? You find that we purchase all other types of food, but we barely think of buying fruits. The good thing about fruits is that they are healthy, and they have plenty of nutritious benefits. If you are the type of person that loves sweet things, fruits can act as a good replacement. When consumed, they add value to your body and can prevent you from acquiring some diseases.

Avoid processed foods

Currently, we are having a lot of processed foods. The food industry has been one of the fastest-growing industries. As the industry expands, the market becomes competitive, and more people join the industry. We are having new foods being introduced to the market as companies look forward to growing and gaining recognition.

One of the common factors among all the companies is that they aim at pleasing the consumers. After carefully studying the target market, they know what each individual requires, which helps them in the production of their various items. If they are targeting a market with low purchasing power, they make products that are cheap and enticing. Some of the processed foods made by such companies contain a lot of chemicals and have harmful effects on the individual.

You find that such foods are not helpful and only result in harm. These are the types of foods that we need to avoid if we wish to have good health. One of the things that you require for you to avoid such foods is discipline. It allows you to make the right decisions regarding what you consume, and you only take in what is helpful.

Avoid carbohydrates

In every meal that you take, you only require a small portion of carbohydrate. In most cases, we do the contrary and have the biggest percentage of our meal as a carbohydrate. When we go to this, our body receives more that it can utilize. One of the main purposes of consuming carbohydrates is that they provide us with energy. When they are consumed in excess, not all can be used to provide energy. The excess can be turned into fatty tissues, and one ends up adding some weight. In some cases, the carbohydrates can result in some diseases like cardiovascular diseases.

To avoid weight gain and such diseases, it is better if one avoids taking large amounts of carbohydrates. Ensure that you only take the recommended portions. You also find that some of these foods, like bread, contain certain addictive substances. In the process, all you want to do is keep wanting to take more. As a result, you take up more than your body needs, and the excess does not benefit it in any. Mediation can help you attain some self-control. You get to eat the amount of food that your body requires.

Eating the recommended portion of food

Eating right can mean taking the amount of food that one needs. You find that certain chronic eating disorders prevent us from eating as we should. An individual with bulimia tends to consume more food than the required portion. There are various factors that can cause an individual to do so. For instance, they might be struggling with low self-esteem due to how they look. Some petite individuals wish they were a little bit bigger. As a result of their esteem issues, they end up consuming more than the required amount of food.

There is a certain belief within them that if they eat a lot, they will get to the size they want. Sadly, that is not always the case. At times their body experiences no change, which can cause an individual to be frustrated. The same applies to eat less than the required amount of food. Skipping some meals is not good. You end up causing more harm to your body when you should be taking proper care of it. The best thing to do is to ensure that you take the recommended amount. This ensures that you stay healthy and fit. With the aid of mediation, you can maintain focus.

Consuming plant-based meals

Everyone should turn to eat vegetables. Plant-based meals contain nutrients that are helpful to our bodies. Some of the minerals present to ensure that our bodies are functioning as they should, and normal body processes are being conducted well. The nutrients are effective in ensuring that we maintain good health by providing minerals that prevent certain diseases. Some of these minerals help in boosting the various metabolic processes occurring in our bodies. In case you have not been consuming plant-based meals, you have been missing a lot. Plant-based meals are also effective in weight loss. They ensure that we take only the right food portion that is helpful to our bodies. When most people want to start a weight loss journey, the immediate solution is talking plant-based meals. They have proven to be beneficial in that journey and process. In the past, people used to live long and were healthy because of consuming such diets. At this time, people would eat what they planted or what they hunted. They ate right and led a healthy life. One needs some discipline for them to eat plant-based meals.

Eat lightly cooked food

When we overcook meals, they do not have nutritious benefits to our bodies. You find that all the nutrients that were present are lost in the process. As you consume that food, it is not helpful to your body. Foods are beneficial when raw or when lightly cooked. Not everyone might manage to eat the foods when they are in this state. One needs some certain level of discipline for them to lightly cook their food and consume it in that state. At times you find that it is easier to consume food when fully cooked, especially with the taste that comes with it. You want to eat something sweet and something that you can easily chew. The problem with such desires is that the food will not help you in any way. At times you are torn between enjoying your meal or eating right. The two are difficult choices to choose from, and you may find yourself opting to enjoy your meal. Eating healthy can be fun, only if you tune your mind into it. Meditation will help you maintain focus, and you will easily accomplish the goals that you have set.

Reduce your sugar intake

Sugars are sweet and enticing. They make you want to eat more, and you simply cannot have enough of them. At times you crave to eat something that is sweet to your taste buds. The problem is the effect that these sugars have on your body. You find that when you consume them in excess, they cannot be utilized by the body. Instead of being converted into energy, they are converted into fats. When this happens, it can result in further complications to your body.

We have some diseases such as diabetes that result from consuming excessive sugars. We also have some challenges, such as tooth problems that result from consuming sugars. At times they can be addictive, and all we wish to do is to take more of them. However, with the right discipline, we can regulate our sugar consumption. You can decide that you will be taking only a certain amount of sugars in a day. Meditation allows you to be focused on what you do. In this case, your focus is on regulating the number of sugars that you take. With this, you get to consume that which is necessary. In the end, it ensures that you have good health and that your body is in the right shape

Avoid overeating

Overeating is a bad eating habit that everyone should avoid. In the process of overeating, one gets to add extra weight, and it has some harmful effects on their body. Mindful eating is essential in ensuring that we maintain good health. An individual's ability to focus can help them know when they are full. Different foods have different food components. There are some foods that will make you feel full at a fast rate than others will. You can analyze how your body feels after eating certain types of foods and know the effect of each food.

This analysis helps you determine the portion that you should consume depending on the type of food involved. As a result, you make better and more informed decisions in terms of what you consume and watch the quantity that you take. To effectively follow this, one requires self-control that ensures they stick to the plan.

This may appear like a challenging thing to accomplish, but it is possible with the help of meditation. You only need to tune your mind into consuming that which is necessary.

CHAPTER 8:

Stop Emotional Eating

Understanding the Causes of Emotional Eating

When you're stressed or frustrated, you tend to look for chewy or crunchy foods like cookies or candy bars. When you're feeling sad, lonely, or depressed, you tend to look for soft or creamy textured foods like ice cream or chocolate.

Sadness, loneliness, and depression reflect a lack of love and attention.

When you pay attention to the pattern of eating, you will notice the difference between the two types of eating. Once you identify what is leading you to desire to eat, you can take care of what you need instead of looking for it in food.

This is not the blanket one to identify the connection. It may not work for everyone. There are times you won't identify the specific need that you have but keep searching. Eventually, you will know the exact connection between food and the emotions to a certain degree of accuracy.

Pressure emotions; anger, frustration or resentment

The cravings are for a specific food. You know exactly what you want. The craving is so precise that you can go to the food store to get a specific brand of cookies or nuts. You do what it takes to satisfy the food thought, including getting up in the night to get a bag of French fries.

Foods that you crave when you are frustrated often include nuts, French fries, chewy, meat, hot dogs, pizza or crackers. These foods provide the chewiness or crunchiness that requires an effort to give the feeling of satisfaction. It replaces the thought of having to express the frustration or anger to somebody else. Instead, you direct it to food.

Managing Pressure Emotions

When you feel the intense urge to eat chewy or crunchy foods, reflect on what is bothering you. What exactly is irritating or stressing you? Is it that your job is difficult, and you are using food to make it through the day?

Stress, deadlines, and people are a common reason for this eating. When you feel the pressure building, you use food as a quick way to relieve the tension as quickly as possible. Food always seems like the fastest and easiest way than doing yoga or listening to music.

Be honest about how you feel and avoid facing the emotions. Once you identify the cause of how you feel, ask yourself if eating will solve the issue. Will food take away the root cause of the problem?

Will food push over the deadline or remove your stressful boss? If you keep eating, you will get stuck in the same pattern that you desperately want to fix. Eating may seem to solve the problem because you feel better after you eat. But after a few hours, the issue you're running away from will still be there and cause you to eat again. It merely postpones what you should do.

Take the issue heads on and tackle the issue. If it is beyond you, try simple ways to relax like taking a short walk or listen to music. List down activities that you can do on what to do as soon as you start feeling these emotions before your mind shifts the focus to eating.

When you get a food craving due to these emotions, do just one for the favorite responses that you have selected. Give yourself about ten minutes before you eat anything. These activities may not solve the issue, but they will give your mind time to reflect.

Rather than reaching out for food, think about the root cause of the emotion you're feeling and address it.

Don't fall for the temptation to eat a little bit; you may not manage to stop at one bite.

Feelings of sadness, loneliness, hurt, yearning for love and depression

These feelings make you feel empty, bored, discouraged, depressed, and alone. They don't provoke a specific food craving but push you to eat 'comfort foods.' You wander around the house wanting to eat something, but you don't know what to eat.

You are unsure of what food will feel good for that moment. But you know you want to eat something. When you chose what to eat, you often go for soft and creamy textured foods like ice cream, pies, milkshakes, cake, and pasta. These foods provide a soothing effect and relate to memories of happy times.

The emotions make you yearn to eat what is missing in your life, like love, attention, or appreciation. When emotions come, you eat sweet and smooth foods like cake, ice cream, or sweet foods. Many happy moments are when we eat sweet foods. As a child you probably were comforted with sweet when you cried, so you get hooked to sweets as an adult to recoup the memories where you felt comforted and nurtured.

When lonely and anxious, it pushes you to look for something familiar and comforting in food. People eat through all kinds of challenges to get the comfort that food offers. You yearn to get a hug, to be nurtured and comforted. But since you may be all alone, food offers the comfort just temporarily.

Managing These Emotions

Whenever you feel the urge to eat, but you don't know what, reflect on what is happening at that moment. What is prompting your desire to eat? What need do you have? Probably you need a friend, or you have experienced a difficult time, or your life feels boring, and you felt there is something you're lacking.

Ask yourself if eating will change your situation. You may get the short-term soothing and comfort that food provides, but the emotion will still come back if you don't handle the root cause of your feelings. You will still have to deal with the real challenge after the comforting feeling of food wears off. Food temporarily hides the pain, but it doesn't make it disappear.

The best way to handle these emotions is to come up with a list of activities that you can do instead of reaching out for food. The activities include reading, listening to music when you feel sad, or taking a class or a hobby when you feel bored. You can also take a hot shower or soak in the bathtub. Do something nice for yourself like going for manicure or pedicure. Also, consider volunteering at children's home or the elderly home where you can get hugs, and as you comfort others, you will also be comforted. You can also stroke or hold an animal or a stuffed animal.

Most times, you crave a particular food because it reminds you of a time when your needs were met in the past. You eat as a way to recapture the old feelings of happiness prompted by your memory.

Don't wait before everything is perfect before you make changes in your life. You can stop the emotional eating patterns right now and start on a positive way of handling emotions. Any time you feel the urge to eat, ask yourself what the exact issue is. Always remind yourself that food will never solve your problem.

Why We Eat

We should eat to provide our body with nourishment and energy. But we eat for many other reasons. We eat the way we do because of our culture and how we were brought up. We eat out of habit or to satisfy expectations from our peers. Other times we eat in response to our emotions, whether to calm down anger or to comfort us. We also eat from compulsion or as a reward.

The primary reason for eating should be to satisfy the physical hunger, which is the body's way of getting the fuel it needs to function throughout the day. In our current fast-paced society, our intake of food is much greater than we need. Our level of activity is nonexistent. Everything has been made easy to achieve. At work, we labor in our desks until dawn. When we get home, the ease of remote-controlled gadgets keeps us on the couch as we watch TV, dim the lights or close the curtains. The result is that we are suffering from the choices that we have made.

The effect of culture on how we eat

Our culture determines our relationship with food. It determines how we combine foods and how we eat food. Some cultures embrace vegetarianism, while others eat more animal meats than plant-based diets. Some cultures place importance on sharing meals and eating together.

The cultural norms play a huge role in the relationship that you have with food. List down some food cultures you can remember growing up so that you can discover the relationship you have with food. List how you can still practice your culture without affecting your relationship with food.

Childhood experiences with food

As adults, we eat just the same way our parents or guardian taught us. Try to remember what food patterns you learned as a child and ho it has impacted your life as an adult.

Some practices include cleaning up your plate. If it was wrong to leave some food on your plate, and you could not leave the dinner table before you finish your food as a child, you will find that as an adult you may overeat so that you don't pour food.

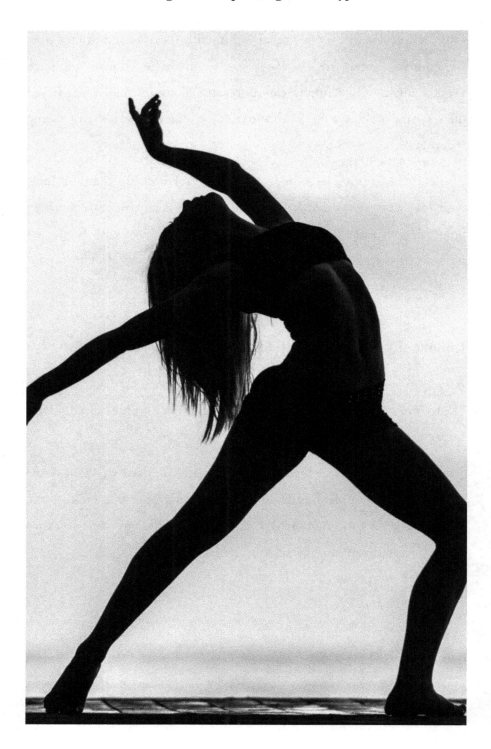

CHAPTER 9:

Step to Avoid Emotional Eating

I f you want to gain control over your life and stop emotional eating, you need to understand a few basic things. Firstly, it cannot be done in a single day just because you suddenly say you will stop eating that way. The problem is deep-rooted and will require some effort, but it's not impossible. Don't think of it as something too easy or too difficult. The first step is to identify the problem and then you can start dealing with it. It won't be a single step toward a healthier you but an entire process that will help you with. As you go step by step, you will slowly be able to stop eating unless you are truly hungry, and you will learn how to deal with your emotions in a healthier way.

Diagnosis of Emotional Eating

Many different health care providers or specialists help to evaluate and treat emotional eating. Over the years it has become a much more prevalent problem than it was a couple of decades ago. Emotional eating is a major contributing factor to obesity and excessive weight gain in people, and this has made professionals more aware of the need to deal with the problem. When you know that the problem is serious, it is best to consult a professional for help. You might need a consultation with a psychologist, help from a pediatrician, or monitoring of your eating. Sometimes just one doctor is enough to help you out, but for those who deal with a more severe problem like an associated eating disorder, multiple sources might be required.

The initial diagnosis of emotional eating is made after a proper physical examination and tests to check for any medical conditions or genetic factors. There are some standardized tests with questions for the patient to answer in order to assess the condition. The patient's mental health history is studied to check for eating disorders like pica or bulimia or any mental illnesses. All this together is used to determine whether the person suffers from emotional eating and the extent of it.

Identifying the Triggers of Emotional Eating

You need to start by identifying what triggers you to start eating when you're not even hungry. Think about the last few times you had sudden cravings or binged on food. Write these instances down on a list. Seeing it written down can be quite revealing and help you see the pattern of ignoring problems and eating to combat them. There can be many different reasons for emotional eating. To deal with your emotional eating, you must identify what triggers it. What kinds of situations, people, or feelings make you want to eat your comfort foods? Do you eat when you feel sad to drown your sorrows? Or do you eat when you want to celebrate an event? Does being around a particular person make you want to indulge in food to feel better? Everyone has different triggers, so don't shrug off a reason just because it seems normal to you. Some people are triggered when they are stress about work. You might be emotionally eating when you have to do something you didn't want to. You might compulsively eat every time you see food or pass by a food stall. Maybe you eat every time you think of or hear about a particular food, or you feel obligated to eat just because you know its lunch or dinnertime and can't seem to skip it even if you're not hungry. You might just keep eating whenever you're bored and have nothing to do. Some people eat more when they are stressed by the people around them, like relatives at a family gathering. All of these and many more could be triggers for your unhealthy emotional eating habits. Until you identify them, you cannot start to overcome the habit.

Ideally, everyone would eat only when they were hungry and only as much as their body really needed. We would all be able to stop eating as soon as our stomach was full and not hungry anymore; however, most of us eat a lot when affected by extrinsic factors like being part of a celebration or when dealing with stress. This is why you need to work on building a healthy relationship with food. Your attitude should be one of "eat to live" rather than "live to eat." Appreciating food is very different from being obsessed with it. An unhealthy relationship with food can be the root of many problems, both physically and emotionally. Identifying the triggers for your eating will make you more conscious of your actions in the future. You will become more aware of what you are doing every time you reach for food. Once you know your triggers, you have a better chance of dealing with them.

Understanding Your Reasons

Once you have written down all the triggers that lead to your emotional eating, try to understand why they affect you negatively. It may have seemed completely normal to eat that way in some situations, but when you compare your behavior to others', you will see the issue. For instance, if you go to a birthday party, it might seem compulsory for you to eat the cake, but your friend might say no. At that time, you probably thought it weird for them to refuse cake since it's a basic part of the occasion, but now that you question it, you realize it's just a conditioned habit and that you don't really have to eat it if you don't want to. The problem is that you never stopped to think about it and just ate the cake because it was there.

Start looking at the list of your triggers and question why each one affects you. Write down the answers beside the list. Don't write answers like "it's normal," but instead think about what makes you want to indulge in emotional eating in the moment of that particular trigger. Keep questioning yourself till you realize how you linked that particular situation to eating over the years.

Detach These Triggers from Food

After all the self-questioning, you know most of the reasons behind why these triggers prompt you to eat. The next step is to work toward disassociating food from these triggers. Try to understand how each link was established. At some point in the past, you started eating in response to a particular situation, and over time your body became conditioned to it. You need to identify what that situation was and accept that this link you established is not really normal and is very different from how other people react to the same situation. If you want to stop yourself from continuing the same self-destructive behavior, you first have to accept that it is not healthy and is incongruent with how others deal with situations.

Once you start accepting that it was wrong to link eating with those triggers, you will start understanding that it was all in your mind. In reality, the triggers don't have any relation to eating, and you shouldn't link them in that way. The triggers have to be separated from the eating since the two things are completely different issues. Eating should be linked only to physical hunger that has to be satisfied to provide the body with energy. The triggers that cause emotional eating are completely irrelevant to why you should eat.

For instance, think about how you associate food with celebrations. You will see that most celebrations in the past have had a lot of food involved. Thanksgiving tables are always filled with food, and everyone eats till they're stuffed and not just till their hunger is sated. As kids, we went to fast food places like McDonald's right after exams were over to celebrate with sodas and burgers. As adults, we treat ourselves to a fancy restaurant dinner when the paychecks come in. Celebrations have always been deemed incomplete without a lot of food to enjoy them with. This is why our brains are synced to associate food with celebrations every single time, but you need to realize that it's a very illogical way of thinking. Why do you need to eat excessive food to celebrate something good? It's not just the fact that you eat unhealthy food but also how much more you eat than necessary.

Another example is dealing with cravings. Sudden cravings for food are one of the most common symptoms of emotional eating. Most of the time, these cravings are associated with junk food or any unhealthy food that gives you a momentary rush. When you have such cravings, you might think that it's a form of hunger and you absolutely have to satisfy it, but you need to start thinking about these cravings more and realize that they are linked only to your mind and not your body.

If you stop and ask yourself why you keep craving a particular food, you will understand better. Most of the time it's because you associate that food with something good that happened and eating it makes you feel better again. There are certain foods like pancakes or waffles that your mom might have treated you with when you were younger. As you grow older, eating these things imparts a sense of comfort and goodness in you again, but if you think about it, you felt good because of your mother and not the food. The food was just one way she showed you love, but it was not the root of it. If you want to feel better in a situation, think about her and not the food.

Deal with The Triggers

Emotional eating usually happens when you don't want to deal with a certain emotion or situation. In order to turn off this trigger, you need to first deal with it. Eating cannot act as a makeshift solution. If you don't deal with the problem and try to resolve it, it won't go away. Eating will just suppress your emotions and help you push the problem to the back of your mind. You might feel better and not think of it for a while, but it will continue to come forward until you actually resolve it. Because emotional eating is largely associated with stress, one of the most crucial aspects of this is stress management. As you read on, stress management will be dealt with in a more thorough manner to help you through it.

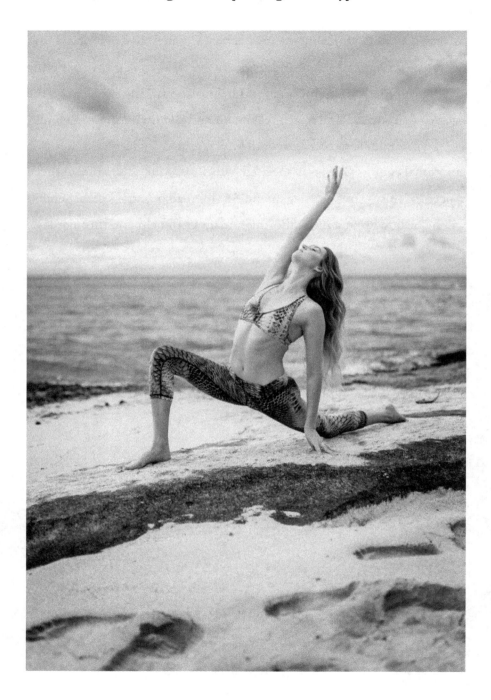

CHAPTER 10:

Deal with you Emotions Without Using Food

First, abandon the idea that your emotional diet is terrible or uncontrollable. Not as much as most people do. Outside the context of food culture, we can even argue that raw food not slandered as it is now. We go to the point where emotional meals are useful.

An emotional diet is a way to let your body know something is wrong. It's pretty smart when you think about it. It's a clue, and it's a way for your body to tell you something is happening, and you need to deal with it. It is a coping mechanism.

Food is closely related to emotions from a very young age. When the baby cry, parents provide them with milk. When you are a kid and won a dance contest, you go to celebrate pizza. There are cakes at birthday parties and weddings—ice cream when I broke up with my boyfriend.

When we are sad, funerals have sandwiches and sausage rolls. Using food to relieve unpleasant emotions is not inherently wrong. It's probably healthier than going home with a man who doesn't remember the name because of a blind drunk (don't say some of us weren't there!)

I'm concerned when food (or lack of food!) Is your only coping mechanism: if you don't know other ways to handle emotions, limit your dietary intake to deal with it

A note on emotional overeating or restriction: For many people, the tendency to be unresponsive when faced with difficult or challenging emotions. In many ways, this reaction is similar to eating to relieve negative emotions. Emotional overeating and overeating are both ends of the same spectrum.

In many cases, when people eat snacks in response to difficult emotions, it becomes a form of control. The world around them is messy, unfair, and unpredictable.

However, you can control what you eat and how much. Just as being overfull, the physical sensation of hunger can distract from more painful emotions and help deal with stress. By building an emotional coping toolkit, nourishing the body is one of the essential things we can do to show that we care about ourselves. On the other hand, withholding food can indicate a lack of self-esteem. Returning to the list of 100 things you wrote about yourself, you can recall how wonderful you are. Before that, let's consider what the emotional diet did to help you. I know it sounds strange. For most people, raw food is bad news and is something that you want to close quickly, if not immediately. But here it is. If the emotional diet did not serve an essential purpose, would you have thrown it away? Raw food is not inherently wrong. It might have been the best way to deal with when something painful or difficult happened in life. A maladaptive coping mechanism is just a representation of an unmet need.

If we can try and understand the purpose that emotional meals are useful in your life, we get substantial clues about what your needs are.

Think about when you use food to relieve unpleasant emotions or deal with stressful situations. For example, you may have felt lonely, and food has helped distract you from loneliness or relieve that unpleasant feeling. Perhaps you are dealing with complicated things such as divorce, illness, bereavement, and you needed some sweetness in your life. Maybe you were angry at something, so you had to take it out with some food.

I know this may seem unnatural but go with it. In your diary, write all the functions that numbness, distraction, comfort, and food have played to relieve unpleasant emotions. Write down your reflection along with it. Did this give you a clue about your own unmet needs? For example, if you are unfortunate, maybe the food.

Emotional Hunger Vs. Physical Hunger

Physical hunger: Now that I understand the signs and symptoms of physical famine, I will summarize it for safety.

● Build gradually

● Low energy

● Satisfied by eating something

- I'm hungry/irritated (I feel safe when I eat)

- Time has passed since the last meal or snack

There is also a taste hunger. This is the feeling that you want to eat something just because you like the taste. This is usually met by having two spoons of Nutella or peanut butter, some chips, a bowl of ice cream, some cheese slices, and so on. If you feel you need much more food to satisfy that desire, you may be seeing emotional hunger.

Emotional hunger:

- No physical hunger clues

- Particular craving

- I am not completely satisfied with the food (or I feel I need more food)

- Occurs immediately after the last meal or snack

- I'm looking at the refrigerator/kitchen

If you have confirmed that you are not 100% physically hungry, hungry, and not full of food, you may be experiencing emotional hunger. The tricky part is identifying what you are feeling. This can be difficult if you are used to stuffing instead of feeling, not feeling.

Ask yourself whether the feelings you are feeling are related to your eating desire. Here are some common emotional triggers that help food in that particular situation.

Abandonment-food is always there, and it is a reliable constant in your life

Anxiety – Use food to calm your nerves

Boredom – using the menu as excitement

Committee-"I deserve this because I had a ridiculous day."

Frightened-The food calms you down

Sky – diet helps you fill the emptiness you feel

Inappropriate-creating and preparing food can give you a sense of purpose

Joy – food is a celebration

Pride-"I got this snack because I received a promotion."

Loneliness-food reminds you of happy times with friends and even acts as friends

Sadness – peaceful food makes you happy in the short term – carbohydrates can boost serotonin

Reward – "I got this."

Emotion word wheel

It is difficult to recognize what you are feeling, especially if you are accustomed to using food to numb your emotions. There are two ways to try it according to your mood. The first is to use the circle of emotions in reverse to help put words or words into what you may be feeling. It might be easier to identify the excitement in the middle and narrow it down outward.

The feelings around the outside are a little more subtle.

If it's difficult to name your emotions, you can use the person outline below to identify where you feel in your body. Each emotion has a physical sensation. Like bodily conditions such as sleepiness and natural diet cues such as hunger and fullness, passion is a component of cognitive receptivity. To the outline that feels emotion, it may be in multiple locations. Let's acquire a little creativity. By increasing or decreasing the feeling, you can give it a color, shape, or strength. You can print several outlines to map emotions over time and see if there is a pattern. You can also be aware of whether there were significant events, such as a fight with a partner.

Understanding Body Sensation

Where emotions are in your body, there may be multiple emotions at the same time. For each sense, consider the next dimension or characteristic of emotion. Physical location: head, heart, chest, stomach, shoulder, neck, jaw, lungs, etc.

Shape: Circle, triangle, irregular blob, wavy line, spiral, curved, octagon, etc.

Color: This is entirely subjective. Choose a color that best reflects your emotions

Size: How strong emotions are felt may be reflected in the size

Once you have decided on the shape your feelings will take, draw it in a diagram.

You can see a visual representation of your emotions; can you use a word from the word wheel to name it?

Can you identify the trigger of emotions?

Can you identify what purpose food serves to relieve that emotion?

Does this give you clues about what you need and how to meet your needs?

Conclusion

Albert Einstein believed that a life shared with others is worthy. We have people out there who need you, remember not to hoard your successes.

Share your success. Share your new-found recipes, your attitude, and your habits. Share what you have learned with others. In all your undertakings, know that you can't change other people but yourself, therefore, be mindful. Reflect on your changes and Put yourself on the back today and every day. Be grateful and live your life as a champion.

Make it a reality on your mind the fact that the journey to a healthy life and weight loss is long and has many challenges. Pieces of Stuff we consider more important in life require our full cooperation towards them. Just because you are facing problems in your Wight loss journey, it does not mean that you should stop, instead show and prove the whole world how good your ability to handle constant challenges is — training your brain to know that eating healthy food together with functional exercises can work miracles.

Make it your choice and not something you are forced to do by a third party. Always tell yourself that weight loss is a long process and not an event. Take every day of your days to celebrate your achievements because these achievements are what piles up to massive victory. Make a list of stuff you would like to change when you get healthy they may be Small size-clothes, being able to accumulate enough energy, participating in your most loved sports you have been admiring for a more extended period, feeling self-assured. Make these tips your number one source of empowerment; you will end up completing your 30 days even without noticing.

You have made it, or you are about to make it. The journey has been unbelievable. And by now, you must be having a story to tell. Concentrate on finishing strongly. Keep up the excellent eating design you have adopted. Remember, you are not working on temporary changes but long-term goals. Therefore, lifestyle changes should not be stopped when the weight is lost.

Remind yourself always of essential habits that are easier to follow daily. They include trusting yourself and the process by acknowledging that the real change lies in your hands. Stop complacency, arise, and walk around for at least thirty minutes away. Your breakfast is the most important meal you deserve. Eat your breakfast like a queen. For each diet, you take, add a few proteins and natural fats. Let hunger not kill you, eat more, but just what is recommended, bring snacks and other meals 3- five times a day.

Have more veggies and fruits like 5-6 rounds in 24 hours. Almost 90% of Americans do not receive enough vegetables and fruits to their satisfaction. Remember, Apple will not make you grow fat. Substitute salt. You will be shocked by the sweet taste of food once you stop consuming salt. Regain your original feeling you will differentiate natural flavorings from artificial flavors. Just brainstorm how those older adults managed to eat their food without salt or modern-day characters. Characters are not suitable for your health. Drink a lot of water in a day. Let water be your number one drink.

Avoid soft drinks and other energy drinks, and they are slowly killing you. Drink a lot of water in the morning after getting out of your bed. Your body will be fresh from morning to evening. Have a journal and be realistic with it. Take charge of what you write and be responsible.

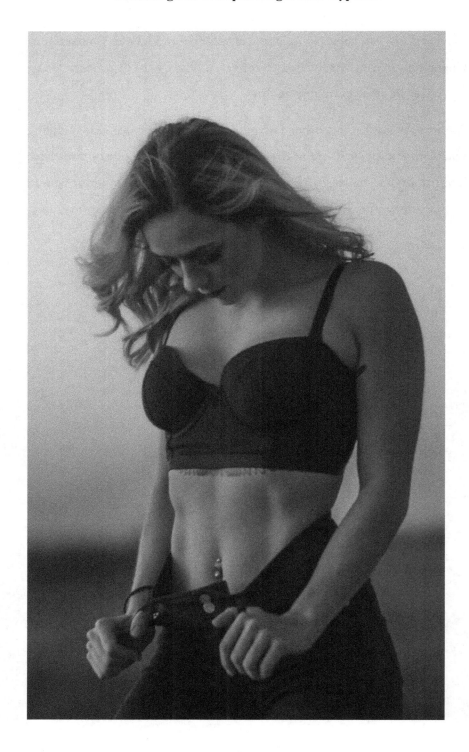

CPSIA information can be obtained
at www.ICGtesting.com
Printed in the USA
LVHW080420010421
683089LV00015B/346